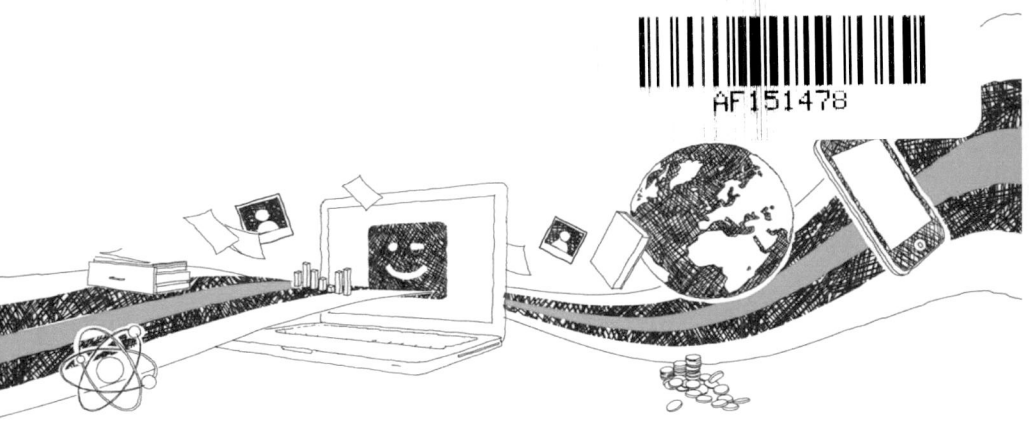
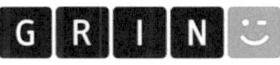

Bibliographic information published by the German National Library:

The German National Library lists this publication in the National Bibliography; detailed bibliographic data are available on the Internet at http://dnb.dnb.de .

Imprint:

Copyright © 2018 GRIN Verlag
Print and binding: Books on Demand GmbH, Norderstedt Germany
ISBN: 9783668659711

This book at GRIN:

https://www.grin.com/document/416037

Patrick Kimuyu

Healthcare Management. Employee Motivation and Motivation Models

GRIN Verlag

GRIN - Your knowledge has value

Since its foundation in 1998, GRIN has specialized in publishing academic texts by students, college teachers and other academics as e-book and printed book. The website www.grin.com is an ideal platform for presenting term papers, final papers, scientific essays, dissertations and specialist books.

Visit us on the internet:

http://www.grin.com/

http://www.facebook.com/grincom

http://www.twitter.com/grin_com

Healthcare Management - Employee Motivation and Motivation Models

Name: Patrick Kimuyu

Introduction

Human beings have brains which respond to various signals in different manners. The nature of the attitude and the ambient environment serve as the principal determinants of an individual appropriate response. Motivation which entails that aspect of acquiring positive attitudes in the surrounding environment and incorporating them into one's behavior, purposely aimed at enhancing performance. Consequently, a motivational behavior appear to be the only influential aspect of human nature that holds promise to realization of one's intended goals in life as an individual. From the work performance perspective, motivation has been known to be a basic tool for improving productivity at the workplace. For this reason therefore, it is important to nature precepts of motivational behavior for profitable output to be realized. In life, individual's strive towards attaining success at last at the end of all tasks that one commits himself/herself ton undertake. On the hand, it is observed that all organizations' main objective is to achieve success. It's absolutely true to assert that all these adorable rewards from any form of work cannot be realized fully if motivation is deficient. In this research paper, all aspects of motivation are going to be discussed for general understanding as well as for identifying the most appropriate ways of nurturing motivational behavior in employees for improved performance at the workplace.

Employee Motivation

At the work place, motivation plays a very fundamental role especially with regard to attitudes of the staff and their employees or rather their managers, who are primarily concerned with supervisory matters to achieve a particular task. Motivation therefore serves as the basic tool at the workplace for managers so as to ensure efficient alignment of aims, values and purpose especially among employees in any organization. Owing to human nature, motivational efforts appear to face a great challenge as each individual possesses personal preferences or attitudes which may be difficult to change or modify (Robbins & Timothy, 2007). As a result, it is important for managers to first identify and comprehend precisely for their employees motivational needs, after which they will take the most appropriate approaches to align their aims and values so as to improve performance hence increased chances of success. Because of this reason, an extensive evaluation of various approaches which have been applied differently by a varied number of managers at different work environment to enhance achieving success.

At the workplace environment, employee motivation has been identified as one of the ingredient for ultimate success. To achieve success, employee motivation skills, motivation models, motivational drives or attitudes as well as expectancy models of motivation have so far been designed.

To produce high quality work, employees require constant motivation either from their own desires to work for the best results possible to be achieved under full commitment or from their leaders and managers. The aspect of motivation of employees at the workplace usually acts as the key determinant factor for success in virtually all organizations. It is therefore great challenge to all managers in charge overseeing the performance of all employees or rather the general staff. Improved productivity at work is recorded when employees are properly given motivation compared to poor results observed when little or no motivation is provided. The principle element of management at all levels lie in employees' motivation. The phrase 'loyal employees' has become common with managers simply because they range productivity of their employees on grounds of performance as well as on their social aspects (Thomas, 2004). Thus it is true that virtually all managers do not value all employees the same. In retrospect, employees are known to have varied attitudes towards their managers depending with the degree of motivation.

Employees' perform at the workplace differ considerably. Subsequently, the overall success of the organization gets affected due to the fact that, in any form of work involving a group of people each with a specific role to play, success depends on their general output. Involvement of a group of individuals in joint execution of a particular task brings in varied human diversity with regard to personality, therefore it has been discovered that the overall success achieved at all times is in one way depended partially on each individual and partially on the collective effort by all individuals. It is important thus to focus on motivation from an individual's perspective and again from the general perspective in the work environment. Owing to these two perspectives, motivation can associated with an individual's personality or as an external influence, that is, from the ambient environment hence the two forms of motivation. Motivation inspired from within an individual is referred to as intrinsic motivation. This type of motivation is believed to be brought about by inherent aspects of a human being such as one's fundamental verities of life, personal goals, happiness, self esteem as well as physiological needs. In other words, intrinsic motivations are attributed to an individual's willingness and desire to achieve a specific goal. On the other hand, motivation inspired from by forces from the surroungding environment is referred to as extrinsic motivation attributed to things that appear to be appealing to an individual. It is actually that aspect of created by as desire to acquire something, or rather that feeling created by the realization that something which you don't have is worth much pleasure. As a result, one sets out to acquire. Desire by every human being to live happily forces one strive for it day-by-day all throughout the entire life because people detest sadness in life. Extrinsic motivation come from such things as; money, prizes, excellent performance results and from other people around you.

An example of intrinsic motivation is seen when an employees does things freely from own preferences and interests. Likewise, some employees show an outstanding interest or passion in their duty or the willingness to learn new skills through real life experience with the main aim of reaching success. On the other hand, employees tend to improve their work efficiency when they are offered incentives.

Motivation Models

Extensive study which has been carried out by a group of psychologists, independently at various time frames and work environment has subsequently designed useful motivational models. These models give a structured guide as the masterpiece of combined effort by individual psychologists particularly on employee motivation. Consequently, various approaches have been designed to address the enormous number of challenges affecting the employees' performance and satisfaction. An overview on motivational models general features was given by the early models developed by two renowned psychologists; G. R. Oldham and Richard Hackman. These old days psychologists explained in details about what they ultimately identified as the fundamental components to motivation, not only in regards to the employees motivation but generally on all aspects of success in life as a whole. Basically, they were driven by such aspects of aims, values and social alignment at the workplace aimed at achieving organizational intended objectives. From the work ethic perspective, they explored on many factors, both intrinsic and extrinsic, and subsequently outlined the basic elements of motivation. For instance, they sought for initiatives that can serve the challenging hurdle of lack of meaningfulness to work, results ownership and the feedback responses. These fundamental elements useful at the workplace identified as: task identity, task significance, skill variety as well as feedback and autonomy.

Skills variety which entails use of different skills and the task identity based on self actualization of the underlying personal potential at the workplace were identified key to enhancing meaningfulness to work. Moreover, the task significance element was also cited to be concerned with enhancement of meaningfulness to work. On the other hand, autonomy was identified to be the only principal element that can enhance employees' ownership of work related results whereas the element of feedback gives an immediate response about the obtained results.

Alternatively, employees' work performance and satisfaction can be boosted significantly through improvement the overall work environment or rather the general structure/features of a particular task. This approach involves incorporation of the five main elements of employees' motivation. These approaches seem to influence the outcome of a single, several or even all of the fundamental elements of motivation. Some of the designed approaches are; first, creating feedback channels: this approach enhance feedback response about the work results. The second approach is building an efficient client relationship so as to increase autonomy, skill variety and feedback altogether. Thirdly, employees' performance and satisfaction can be enhanced through task combination which creates diversity at the workplace, that is, skill variety as well as task identification. Moreover, designing work units influence task identity and task significance to a greater extend. Fourthly, autonomy, task significance, task identity and skill variety can be boosted significantly by providing employees with a high degree of responsibility and ultimate control over the task being undertaken (Carla, 2008).

Specific Models of Employee Motivation

Traditional Theory 'X' (Sigmund Freud's theory)

Sigmund assumed that human beings are absolutely pessimistic with negative attitudes towards work thus he attributed this attitude with the observed tendency by many people to neglect work. He portrayed people as irresponsible, none ambitious and sluggard who seek for cheap means of fulfilling their needs without much struggle. He argued that for people to do any productive work they must be persuaded or rather enticed with such things as rewards or else they can be forced to carry out a given task through harsh treatment by their managers. This has become to be known as the "stick and carrot "philosophy of management. This approach has been proven inconsistent and virtually inapplicable at the workplace where the main goal is to achieve success.

Precisely, this theory does not bring any positive returns because employees are not motivated appropriately to take control of theirs work.

Theory "Y" (Douglas McGregor's Theory)

In retrospect, McGregor refuted the precepts of theory 'X' by claiming that people take work as life obligation: the reasons why they strive tirelessly do achieve meaningful work results. As such, they appear more motivated by their own attitudes which he described as self discipline and self development. Out of his divergent perspective, he viewed the employees' control over their work as being the major aspect that enable employees at work to overcome all odds to achieve optimal efficiency thus improved productivity; contrary to Sigmund's claim that employees enhance their performance at work primarily because they intend to satisfy their desires of receiving cash payment as rewards of their dedication and labor. Theory 'y' therefore appears to consider the manager's role as passive. It allows for uninterrupted self development where the main objective aims at increasing self actualization and gradual attainment of control over work. It is true to assert that the role management now rests on the employees since every member of the organization takes responsibility ultimately pushing forward the basic goals of the organization. Consequently, success at work becomes the ultimate reward of collective responsibility. Respectively, a general growth of all people is also realized (Accel, 2001).

Theory 'Z' (Abraham Maslow's theory)

Abraham's theory is generally a redesigned version of Sigmund's theory; his fellow psychologist. He significantly corrected the classical assumptions brought forward by Sigmund in theory 'X' which where absolutely empirical, that is, they were proven to be unpractical in real-life. Abraham's intuitive revision gave theory 'X' a perpetual change of meaning. He effectively achieved actual results seemingly because he based his line of argument on the human basic needs thus his postulation of the 'hierarchy of needs theory. Abraham argued that people survive primarily on their devotion to work. In addition, he stated that work forms part of a man's life thus having a considerable role in one's overall personality. Moreover, Abraham's opinion on the importance of mans labor closely relate to McGregor's theory especially through his 'Theory of Human Motivation' which highlights various human needs such as need for self-esteem, safety needs, love needs, as well as physiological and self-actualization needs. In other words, he attributed man's work efficiency as a result of the principal wish to fulfill the 'unsatisfied needs'.

Motivation Hygiene Theory (Frederick Herzberg's Theory)

Herzberg's theory attributes work accomplishment to employees' mental health. It is based on both hygiene factors ('animal needs') as well as on human needs (motivators). Herzberg stated categorically that these hygiene factors and motivators as the most important for employee satisfaction.

Expectancy Theory of Motivation (Victor Vroom's Theory)

Organizations require the valuable input from employees so as to have any task done irrespective of whether it produces positive returns or negative. As such, employees are therefore the functional assets of the any organization thus it is important to devise means through which their full potentials can be harnessed for meaningful work output. Relatively, Completion of any Work entirely depends on employees' performance. Performance in turn may be low, moderate or high. It is therefore mandatory for managers to establish employees' performance determinant factors. Motivation drives are ought to be developed on the basis of work-practice, that is, real-life experience for the sake of effectiveness and flexibility owing to the work force diversity. This is however, somehow based on the ever-changing trends of modernity and varied degrees of 'want' by a particular individual at the workplace. In the past, employees' motivational drives have been developed in consideration of rewards and threats, although their needs may require some motivational initiatives which have long been used by managers to enhance employees' performance hence realization of good work results.

By Victor Vroom's perspective, people's decision-making as well as general leadership approaches to various aspects of human nature depend on the ultimate level of expectancy. In other words, he assumed that one's overall character or rather personality is defined by the preferred choices that somebody selectively decides to follow as the most suitable alternatives from an enormous list of possible alternatives. Nevertheless, the preferred alternatives are singled out from the entire list specifically on the intended purpose in one's life, that is, an individual aims at minimizing suffering while maximizing pleasures in life. Vroom's theory as it appears is of strong superstitious nature since all of its major elements are thought to represent a belief of its kind.

However, expectancy theory as developed by Victor Vroom seems offer a very important and reliable tool to address matters of motivation and management altogether.

This theory comprises of three fundamental principles notably, Expectancy (E), Instrumentality (I), and Valence (V). Vroom argues that personality, knowledge, skills/experience as well as personal abilities determine their performance at work. Argumentatively, in agreement with Vroom's point of view it seems a sincere truth that employees' performance is usually directly proportional to their inherent and acquired abilities. He further claimed that all that which we achieve in whatever type of work is determined by our ultimate power to believe that our tireless efforts are correlated to our performance which in turn dictates the magnitude of the rewards obtained at the end. He also observed that the obtained reward fills one's crucial immediate need. Relatively, employee's expectancy at the work place requires one to consider all factors significant and with equal relevance, then it is possible to make consistent attempts that at most incidences lead to excellent performance. Precisely, the power of believing that things can be done and there after reap great benefits from the work results. Simply the impact of positive mental attitude is what makes all to happen after selfless determination to reap meaningful results. Concurrently, the expectancy theory of motivation holds that interaction between expectancy, instrumentality and valence brings about a magnificent psychological outcome or rather a motivational forward spirit to enable an employee to choose the most appropriate alternative way aimed at minimizing pain while receiving maximum pleasures most attainable.

To summarize Vroom's theory of expectancy, it is important to analyze the three basic components that give it all its significance and relevance to both managers as well as to employees collectively. In brief, expectancy entails one's strength to belief that possibilities and impossibilities are fairly expected as final outcomes of any task. Instrumentality on the other hand is based on probability that if someone does a specific task, there are desirable rewards to be obtained at the end (Victor, V. 1968). In this regard, Vroom illustrates chances that two possible outcomes are expected: it means that the probability of one outcome occurring is equivalent to the other equally expected outcome not occurring. Precisely, occurrence of one outcome completely excludes the other outcome from occurring. Finally, valence explains an individual's emotional orientations towards the expected reward as an outcome. A positive valent refer to an employee's preference to reward gain or loss.

Conclusion

Conclusively, all the three elements of expectancy motivational theory usually occur in an interplay scenario for them to bring the resulting outcome. Besides, employees' motivation appears to be a powerful tool for building collaborative and productive workforce within the healthcare system.

References

Accel   (2001).   Motivation   theory   and   Practice.   Accel-Team.Com
     http://www.accel-team.com/motivation/index.html. Retrieved 28th Oct; 2011.

Robbins, S., & Timothy A. (2007). *Essentials of Organizational Behavior* (9 ed.). Upper Saddle
     River, NJ: Prentice Hall.

Thomas, J. (2004). *Guide to Managerial Persuasion and Influence.* Upper Saddle River, NJ:
     Pearson Prentice Hall.

YOUR KNOWLEDGE HAS VALUE

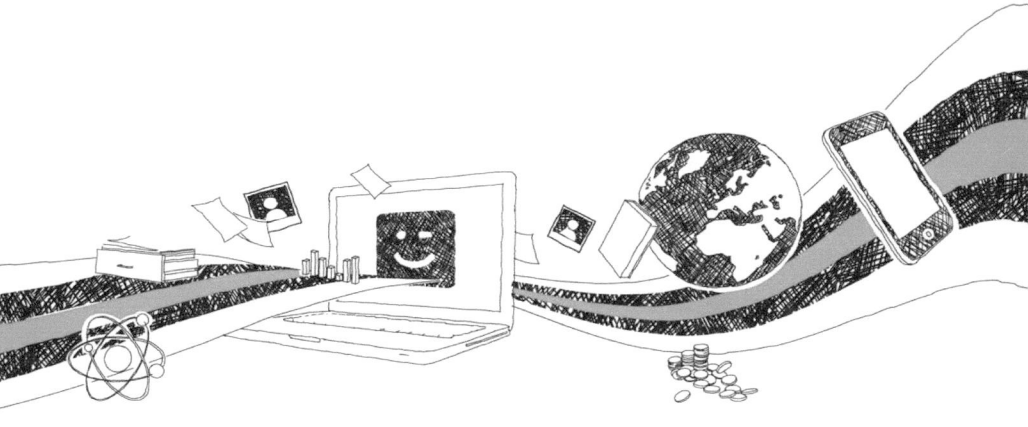

- We will publish your bachelor's and master's thesis, essays and papers

- Your own eBook and book - sold worldwide in all relevant shops

- Earn money with each sale

Upload your text at www.GRIN.com and publish for free

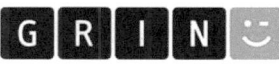